Life's Too Short *for*
TANTRIC
SEX

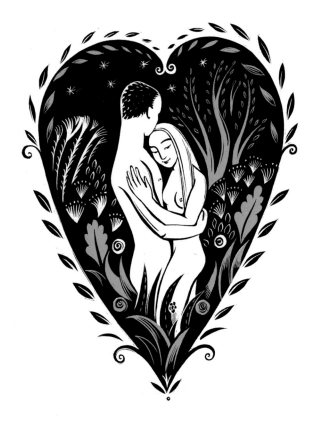

Life's TOO Short *for*
TANTRIC SEX

50 Shortcuts to SEXUAL ECSTASY

KATE TAYLOR

Illustrations by SARAH YOUNG

MARLOWE & COMPANY
New York

LIFE'S TOO SHORT FOR TANTRIC SEX
Text © 2003 Ivy Press Limited
Illustrations © 2003 Sarah Young

Published by
MARLOWE & COMPANY
An Imprint of Avalon Publishing Group Incorporated
245 West 17th Street, 11th Floor
New York, NY 10011

This book was conceived, designed, and produced by
THE IVY PRESS LIMITED
The Old Candlemakers
West Street, Lewes
East Sussex BN7 2NZ, U.K.

THE IVY PRESS

Creative Director: *Peter Bridgewater*   Senior Project Editor: *Caroline Earle*
Publisher: *Sophie Collins*   Mac Design: *Richard Constable*
Editorial Director: *Steve Luck*   Illustrations: *Sarah Young*

Library of Congress Cataloging-in-Publication Data

Taylor, Kate, 1971-
    Life's too short for tantric sex: 50 shortcuts to sexual ecstasy / Kate Taylor
        p. cm.
    ISBN 1-56924-446-4
    1. Sex instruction. 2. Sex. 3. Couples–Time management. I. Title.

HQ31.T3175 2003
613.9'6—dc21

9 8 7 6 5 4

Printed and bound in China
Distributed by Publishers Group West

~ CONTENTS ~

~ INTRODUCTION ~

Sex is not an endurance event. We've all heard tales of marathon lovers who can last for eight hours without yawning, pausing, or getting cramps. But have you ever tried to keep going for that long? Really? Trust me—the three-hour, arm-stroking techniques described in most Tantric sex manuals aren't pathways to ecstasy, they're freeways to fatigue. Great sex, wonderful knee-trembling sex, has nothing to do with deadlines or timesheets, but everything to do with technique and control. It's how you do it that matters, not how long you do it for. With the right information on how your body works and what really turns you (and your lover) on, you can have the best sex of your life in the time it takes to say, "Yes, yes, yes!"

Here is your guidebook to fabulous sex that doesn't require taking days off work. In here you'll find surefire shortcuts to Blissville that are designed to press all of your buttons (and your partner's) with effortless ease. There are tricks and tips for every kind of adventure, from kissing to fantasies, arousal to masturbation, that all promise one thing: the hottest pleasure you've ever felt, in the shortest time you've ever spent.

And, of course, you can do all of them for as long as you like. This doesn't mark the death of the Lost Weekend. It marks the birth of the Lust Weekend, where sex comes in 52 flavors and you've got the time and energy to taste them all.

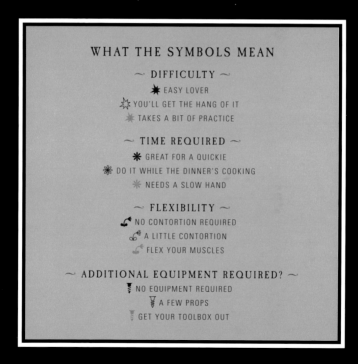

WHAT THE SYMBOLS MEAN

~ DIFFICULTY ~

EASY LOVER

YOU'LL GET THE HANG OF IT

TAKES A BIT OF PRACTICE

~ TIME REQUIRED ~

GREAT FOR A QUICKIE

DO IT WHILE THE DINNER'S COOKING

NEEDS A SLOW HAND

~ FLEXIBILITY ~

NO CONTORTION REQUIRED

A LITTLE CONTORTION

FLEX YOUR MUSCLES

~ ADDITIONAL EQUIPMENT REQUIRED? ~

NO EQUIPMENT REQUIRED

A FEW PROPS

GET YOUR TOOLBOX OUT

SENSUAL MASSAGE
~ for WOMEN ~

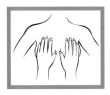

MASSAGES are to arousal what matches are to arson. Come on, boys—start a bushfire.

Make sure the bedroom is comfortably warm. Rub your hands together, and anoint them with lavender, ylang-ylang, or sandalwood massage oil.

Have her lie on her stomach and begin by massaging her scalp and neck with light strokes. Tickle her neck and trace little butterfly kisses over her nape and shoulders. Women's backs are highly erogenous—lick all down her spine while you lightly trace your hands over her ribs. That'll make her ache for you to touch her breasts, but this is not the time. (Not yet. Soon, I promise.) With deeper strokes, using your palms, work up her legs. Kiss the insides of her knees—another hot spot—then massage her inner thighs. When she parts her legs, it's time to turn her over.

☀ EASY LOVER   ❊ DO IT WHILE THE DINNER'S COOKING
     ✍ A LITTLE CONTORTION   ▼ A FEW PROPS

Run the palms of your hands flat over her breasts (I said you wouldn't have to wait long). Pay attention to the area below her nipples—kiss her there for 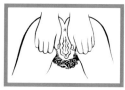 maximum effect. Then lick along her hipbones, working toward her pubic hair. Finally, lubricate your hands with a water-based product like K-Y or AstroGlide, and massage her outer labia with gentle circular thumb strokes. When you've covered every area of her outer lips, gently part them and massage her clitoris. Pull on it—you won't be able to get a proper grip, but it'll feel fabulous. Press both thumbs onto her perineum (the area between vagina and anus) and circle them. She'll feel the vibes all through her body.

Then take it from there. You could just go to sleep of course, but somehow I doubt she'll let you...

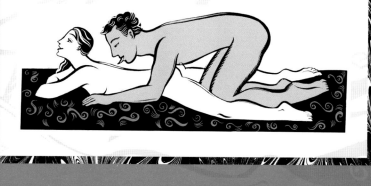

SENSUAL MASSAGE
~ for MEN ~

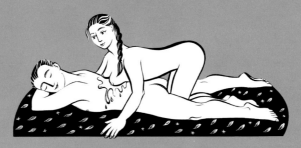

YOU'LL NEED a warm bedroom, some massage oil (try mixing olive oil with cinnamon for a spicy treat), and a wicked side.

Have your man strip naked and lie face down on the bed. Kneel in between his legs, and start by applying the massage oil to your breasts. Then, using slow, gliding movements, caress his back and shoulders with your breasts.

Next, oil your hands and get to work on his buttocks. Place one hand on either cheek and use deep, intense circular strokes. Work

✸ EASY LOVER ✳ DO IT WHILE THE DINNER'S COOKING
⚘ A LITTLE CONTORTION ▼ A FEW PROPS

your thumbs down to his inner thighs, and lightly "graze" them over the underside of his testicles. Part his cheeks and massage around his anus. He'll be a quivering wreck by this time, but don't let up.

Turn him over and press your body against his, working your way down until his penis is between your breasts. Squeeze them together and slide his penis in and out, mercilessly slowly. (If your breasts are too small to accommodate him, rub them over his penis and testicles. It'll feel just as good.)

From there on, the choice is entirely yours. Lick him, suck him, straddle him—or dress him up and have him take you along to Tiffany's. You surely deserve it.

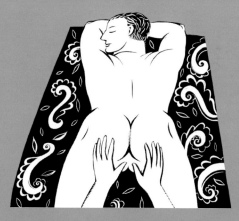

~ *Secret* ~
SEX LANGUAGE

YOUR LOVER will be automatically turned on by some words. All you have to do is discover what they are, and then bam! She'll go to jelly every time you open your mouth. To find out her Secret Sex Language, begin a conversation about fantasies. (A good time is when you're both relaxed after sex.) Encourage your partner to share a recent fantasy she's had. As she talks, listen to her words. More specifically, listen to her "dirty" words—these are the sounds that really turn her on. You might find that she uses words that she would never use in daily life (I couldn't possibly suggest any of them here). Whatever the words, remember them. Then start talking about her fantasy, using those words. Or talk about how you'd next like to make love, using those words. You'll be amazed at the reaction you'll get.

✷ EASY LOVER   **✷ GREAT FOR A QUICKIE**
✫ NO CONTORTION REQUIRED   **⌁ NO EQUIPMENT REQUIRED**

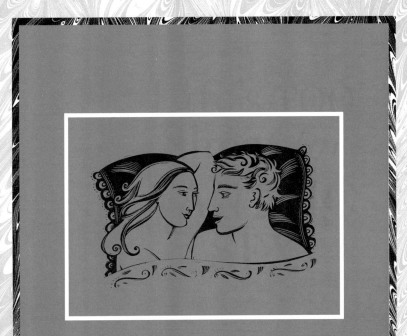

If you are not used to talking dirty (maybe you are not used to talking about sex at all), and feel embarrassed, start off in the dark, or wear blindfolds. That way you can pretend that you are Greta Garbo and John Gilbert, or Sharon Stone and Michael Douglas, or Monica Lewinsky and Bill Clinton—whatever turns you on.

～ LUST *Orders* ～

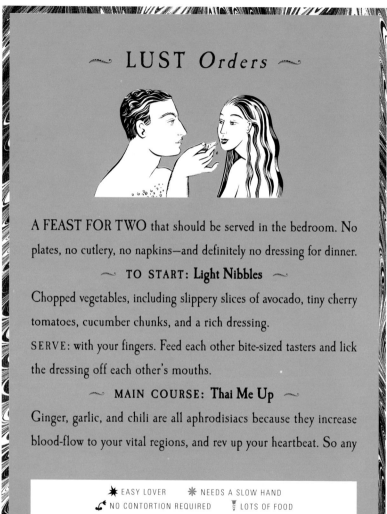

A FEAST FOR TWO that should be served in the bedroom. No plates, no cutlery, no napkins—and definitely no dressing for dinner.

～ TO START: **Light Nibbles** ～

Chopped vegetables, including slippery slices of avocado, tiny cherry tomatoes, cucumber chunks, and a rich dressing.

SERVE: with your fingers. Feed each other bite-sized tasters and lick the dressing off each other's mouths.

～ MAIN COURSE: **Thai Me Up** ～

Ginger, garlic, and chili are all aphrodisiacs because they increase blood-flow to your vital regions, and rev up your heartbeat. So any

✹ EASY LOVER   ✳ NEEDS A SLOW HAND
� NO CONTORTION REQUIRED   ❦ LOTS OF FOOD

kind of curry is recommended. Try Thai dishes, served with sticky rice that you can eat with your fingers.

SERVE: from one dish that you share. Let some of the spicy sauce trickle over breasts and inner thighs, and lick it off.

～ DESSERT: Sweets For My Sweet ～

Strawberries, cream, honey.

SERVE: Drizzle cream over her breasts and lick it off. Pile the halved strawberries on her mound, or arrange them around the base of his penis and nuzzle in. For the finale, cover his penis in honey and make love. The sticky, slightly granular texture of the honey adds friction and can make sex feel incredible.

～ TO DRINK: Champagne, Warm Coffee, Iced Water ～

SERVE: Boys, warm up your mouth with coffee and suck on her breasts, then take a mouthful of iced water and lick her nipples. The warm/cold sensation is HOT.

Girls—fill your mouth with champagne and slide his penis in— the bubbles will tickle more than your tastebuds! Or chill your mouth with iced water and give him a blow job. Then when he is about to come, dip his testicles into the warm coffee. The heat will make him come twice as hard.

The ULTIMATE STRIP

～ WOMEN ～

THERE IS ONLY ONE secret to undressing to impress: confidence. To boost your nerve, have some champagne before you start. Sit him in a chair in front of you, and tell him he that can look but not touch. Put some music on, something with a good bump 'n' grind rhythm (think J Lo or Lenny Kravitz). Wear your sexiest lingerie and pander to his tastes—if he's a black-lace lover, dress like a vamp; if he's a white-panty purist, go innocent. Whichever he is, wear a slip, stockings fastened *underneath* your panties, and high heels.

Once the music starts, look him straight in the eye and start caressing your body over your clothes. Let your hands push the slip up over your thighs, and pull the straps off your shoulders. Step out of it and dance seductively. Next, go right up to him, turn your back and have him unclasp your bra. Turn around, holding your bra on,

✳ EASY LOVER	✳ GREAT FOR A QUICKIE
✒ NO CONTORTION REQUIRED	♟ A FEW PROPS

then let it fall, pushing your naked breasts toward his face. But no touching! Dance away a few steps, and start coyly pushing down your panties. He should feel almost as if he's watching you undress without your knowing, so cast your eyes down and look shy. Then turn your back to him, keep your legs straight, and bend over, pulling the panties off in one go.

Finally, dance over to him wearing just the stockings and high heels, and then sit astride his lap so that he can touch your naked body. Hot? Woman, he'll have scorchmarks.

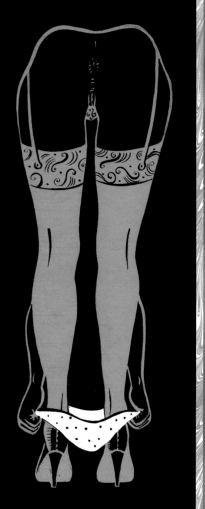

The ULTIMATE STRIP
~ MEN ~

IF YOU'VE SEEN *The Full Monty*, you'll know that women love seeing men ditch their clothes. So here's how to shed the suit without losing your cool (and you don't need any Velcro).

First of all, wear an outfit you know she finds hot. (This is probably your business suit.) But don't wear socks, they're too fiddly to remove. Have her sit on the bed, while you stand opposite her. Put some funky music on, and look her in the eye. Start by loosening your tie, if you're wearing one, and throw it at her. Then slowly, slooooooowly unbutton your shirt, and tear it open. Kick off your shoes, then walk over to the bed and ask her to unbuckle your belt. Then turn around and pull off your pants, giving her a good look at your butt—it's most girls' favorite area!

Last of all are your underpants. Now, most men don't realize how turned on a woman gets by seeing a man touch himself. If you're

---

✳ EASY LOVER   ✳ GREAT FOR A QUICKIE
↝ NO CONTORTION REQUIRED   ⚑ NO EQUIPMENT REQUIRED

one of those men, it's time you learned. Rub yourself through your shorts, until you start getting hard. Then walk over to her and have her pull off your shorts. Whatever happens next is up to you...

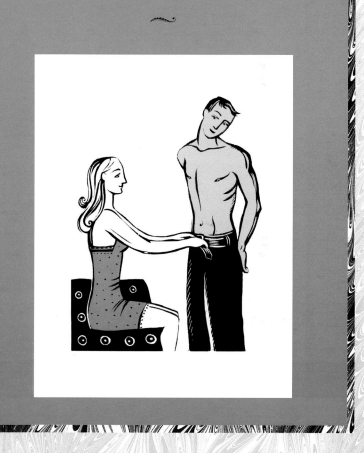

• KISS KISS •

The POWER
~ *of* KISSING ~

THE 30-MINUTE KISS

WHOEVER SAID, "a kiss is just a kiss" was seriously missing a trick. A kiss is much more—it's the ultimate aphrodisiac that can cure libido loss, boost flagging sex drives, and stroke the ego of a flagging penis in moments. The secret is to keep doing it—so many people stop after the third date. So grab your partner, pull him in, and plant a big one on his lips. Really go for it, concentrating all the time on how sexy you can make it. Groan and whimper, dig your fingers into your partner's lower spine, or run your hands, flat, up and down his back. (That works equally well on men and women.) Don't stop for 30 minutes; after that time, your brain will be flooded by a rush of endorphins. And you'll be ready for much more...

~

✳ EASY LOVER ✳ GREAT FOR A QUICKIE
⚷ NO CONTORTION REQUIRED ⚸ NO EQUIPMENT REQUIRED

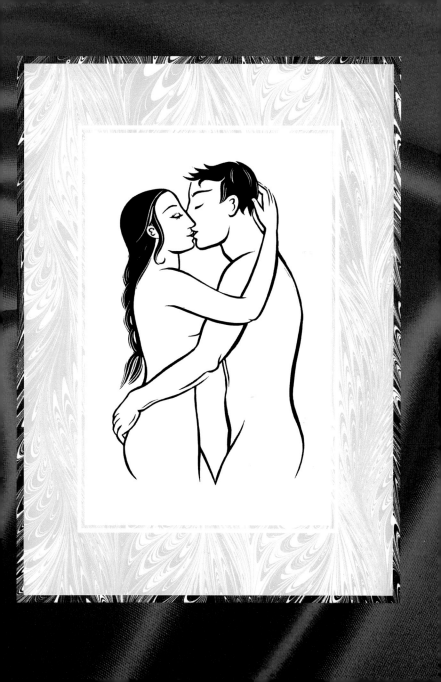

∼ *Where* WOMEN ∼ LIKE *to be* KISSED

THE SECRET to super-sexy kissing is easy: location, location, location. You know that it applies to real estate but it's also how to get her in a real state.

For women, the most erogenous kiss zones are the nape of the neck and along the spine. In fact, these hot spots are rated sexier than mouths for some women. Indian tantra experts believed that was because a "love serpent" lived in women's spines, which uncurled sensuously when it was kissed. It ain't necessarily so, but the reaction you get when you run your tongue down your woman's back might move the animal in you...

Start with some light, butterfly kisses over the nape of her neck. Lick the little bump of bone at the top of her spine, then trail your tongue slowly down her vertebrae. Keep the kisses light—most girls like feathery kisses best. The area right at the base of her spine

❋ EASY LOVER   ❋ GREAT FOR A QUICKIE
  ✄ NO CONTORTION REQUIRED   ⚲ NO EQUIPMENT REQUIRED

is another hot spot, so you'll want to hang around there for a while. Then kiss your way upward again, this time digging your fingertips along her spine (gently please!) as you go. Finally, end with a series of small kisses along her jawline, and then finish on her mouth. Heaven.

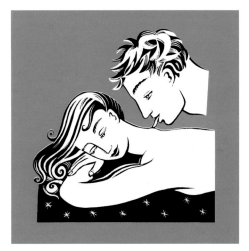

~ *Where* MEN ~ LIKE *to be* KISSED

TO DRIVE A MAN wild with your tongue, don't head immediately due South. Instead, start exploring the very, very sensitive areas above his belt. In fact, above his collar. Men have three truly hot kissing spots: their ears, their neck, and their Adam's apples.

Here's how to ignite them. Start with the ears. Begin nibbling on the lobes, then lick the rim of cartilage that runs around the outer ear. Use your tongue to flick gently inside the ear, making sexy little noises as you go. Then get breathy—but don't blow into the ear. Suck air in, instead. It feels so sexy, like you're turning his brains inside out. (That's a good feeling.)

Next, attack that part of his neck just underneath where his stubble stops; all along that line is super-sensitive. To make him feel more exposed and vulnerable, grasp his hair and pull his head back so his neck is elongated and defenseless. Trace your tongue gently

✷ EASY LOVER   ✷ GREAT FOR A QUICKIE
✺ NO CONTORTION REQUIRED   ⚑ NO EQUIPMENT REQUIRED

along his throat toward his collarbone. Then gently kiss all over his Adam's apple. It's loaded with nerve endings, making it a really erogenous zone, but few women will have kissed him there. You'll be his first—and his last, and his everything.

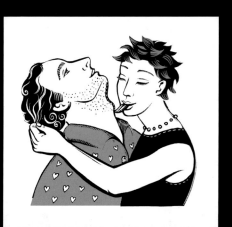

SUCKING
~ *Kisses* ~

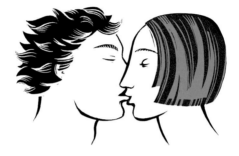

IT'S A VERY BASIC instinct to suck. Just look at babies with mom's nipple or their milk bottles. And when you use the technique in kissing, it awakens primal urges you had no idea you possessed. Try the ancient Honeybee technique.

Using both hands, cover your lover's eyes. This makes him acutely aware of the sensations you're going to give him because he

✳ EASY LOVER   ✳ GREAT FOR A QUICKIE
✄ NO CONTORTION REQUIRED   ⚚ NO EQUIPMENT REQUIRED

can't see what you are doing or where you are going. Start by covering his face in tiny, fleeting kisses like a bee visiting a flower. Next, move down to his mouth and lick his lips until he parts them. Then, gently and slowly, suck on his bottom lip, delicately drawing it into your mouth. Just suck on it very softly for a minute. Run your tongue over it, then lick your way up to his top lip, and suck on that, too. Alternate between his top and bottom lips and then, when he's moaning with desire, suck his tongue into your mouth. Use very gentle, slow sucks—he doesn't want to be in fear of losing his tongue for good—then let go.

You can also suck on his chin, his earlobes, his toes, and his fingers with equally dramatic results. In fact, anything that can be kissed can also be sucked. The only thing that won't suck is you—as a lover. Go on, explore.

～ TONGUE ～
Techniques

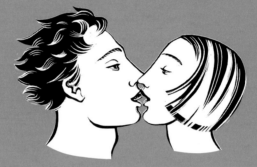

DID YOU KNOW THAT your tongue contains more nerves and muscles in it than almost any other part of your body? This explains why it's the one of the hottest tools that you can use to tantalize your partner—so let's have a workout.

Here's an awesome kissing trick. Start by instigating a long, slow kiss. Part his lips with your tongue, and lick lazily along his bottom

✹ EASY LOVER ✹ GREAT FOR A QUICKIE
ᶜ⸍ NO CONTORTION REQUIRED ⍝ NO EQUIPMENT REQUIRED

lip and his teeth. Then, flick your tongue up underneath his top lip, and lick along his teeth and gums. (While most people adore this, there are some that don't, so do stay aware for clues that he or she is uncomfortable.) Reach your tongue a little farther and lick the roof of his mouth. Some men experience heart failure from this technique so, girls, go careful.

The eyelids are also very rewarding for this sort of kissing. Glide your tongue gently from the outer corner in and back again. Don't press hard—you want your lover to see visions, not have double vision. Once you've finished there, the ears are simply asking to have the soft tip of your tongue slipped into them.

You can also lick the corners of his mouth—two incredibly sensitive spots. While you kiss, imagine you're licking him somewhere else, somewhere far ruder. You'll start using the techniques you would for oral sex, and your partner will quickly pick up on that. Suggestion is a very powerful thing...

KISSING *without*
~ MOUTHS ~

GIRLS, here's an electrifying kissing technique that doesn't involve your mouth at all. You've another pair of warm, soft lips that you can use to kiss him all over his body, and there won't be any lipstick marks... It uses your vaginal lips to "kiss" him all over his body, and it's very, very hot.

During foreplay, when you're both naked, have him lie on his back with his hands underneath him and his eyes closed. Tell him you're going to kiss every area of his body. He'll probably think, "Awww, how sweet," but he's in for a sexy surprise.

Crouch over his body and, making sure that your vulva is wet enough (use some lubricant or saliva if it isn't), start "kissing" him with it. Just squat over him, letting your wet lips press a sexy smacker against his skin. Then start to work down his body, beginning to grind a little deeper with each "kiss." Make sure that you let him

---

✸ EASY LOVER   ✳ DO IT WHILE THE DINNER'S COOKING
⸎ A LITTLE CONTORTION   ⌁ NO EQUIPMENT REQUIRED

know, with your voice, exactly how good it feels whenever you press your clitoris against him. Work your way down to his knees, where you can really rub yourself against him, and then move back up to his penis, and tease him by caressing the tip with your clitoris. Finally, when he can take no more, make love to him.

They call this move the Kiss of Life. Quite apt, because he might need it by the time you've finished with him...

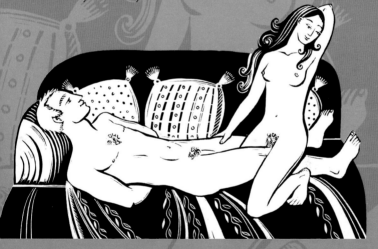

～ *Female* ～
HAND JOB

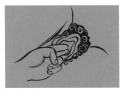

HANDS UP anyone who knows how big the clitoris is. Wrong, wrong, wrong. It's actually very big—equivalent to the size of a penis—extending right around the outer lips of the vagina and down to the urethra. The little clitoral "bud" on the top is only the visible part.

The great thing about this trick is that it can be performed either by a man on his willing partner, or by the woman alone. Rest the heel of your hand on the pubic bone (just below where the hair starts), and hold the outer lips of the vulva open. Pressing down with that hand will start getting some very good vibrations going. Place the index and middle fingers of the other hand on either side of the clitoral bud. Gently start swirling your fingers around and around. The clitoris should be trapped between them, being squeezed as they move.

❋ EASY LOVER   ❋ GREAT FOR A QUICKIE
🌿 NO CONTORTION REQUIRED   🔩 NO EQUIPMENT REQUIRED

All the clitoris is pleasured in this technique, but for heightened stimulation, wet your fingers with lubrication from the vagina, and "tap" the hood that covers the clitoral bud (the clitoris itself is too sensitive for this kind of attention). Combined with the pubic-bone pressure, it feels out of this world.

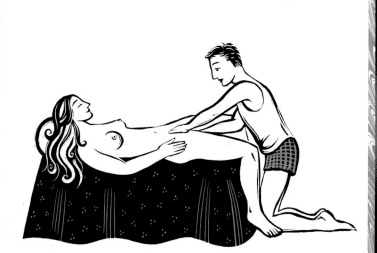

～ ACCESS ～
all AREAS

IT'S NO SECRET that there are four points of maximum joyous potential in and around the vulva: the clitoris, the vagina—especially the G-spot—the perineum (the spot just below the vagina and above the anus), and the anus itself. Although it's great to devote quality one-on-one time to each of these hot spots, sometimes life is indeed too short, and you want a technique that will ring all the bells at once.

Access All Areas requires supple fingers—lucky you if your profession is that of concert pianist or safecracker—and a sensitive touch. It works best if the vagina is already well lubricated. The whole hand is used, left or right. Use the thumb to gently massage the clitoris (start with the hood); at the same time slide index or third finger (or both) into the vagina to stimulate the G-spot on the vaginal wall; and finally use the little finger to massage the perineum or stimulate the anus.

✨ YOU'LL GET THE HANG OF IT   ✳ GREAT FOR A QUICKIE
🐍 NO CONTORTION REQUIRED   ⚡ NO EQUIPMENT REQUIRED

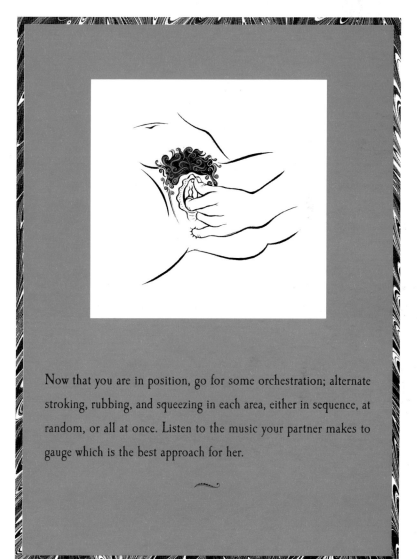

Now that you are in position, go for some orchestration; alternate stroking, rubbing, and squeezing in each area, either in sequence, at random, or all at once. Listen to the music your partner makes to gauge which is the best approach for her.

~ OPEN *Wide* ~

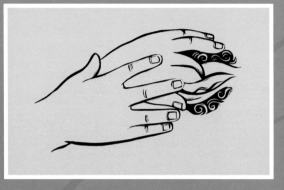

MEN, forget flowers and chocolates. What women really want is the sort of skillful manipulation that has them bouncing off the ceiling. This is such a technique.

Sit upright, with your partner in between your legs, her back against your chest. If you can't reach her vulva comfortably in this position have her sit on a pillow. Begin by caressing her breast with

YOU'LL GET THE HANG OF IT   ✳ GREAT FOR A QUICKIE
A LITTLE CONTORTION   ▼ NO EQUIPMENT REQUIRED

one hand while you keep the other arm around her to hold her close. Circle her nipples softly with your fingertips until you feel she is relaxed and ready. Then place both hands on her belly. Slip two fingers inside her and rub gently on the front wall of her vagina. About two inches up, you should feel a small patch of tissue smoother than the rest—that's her G-spot. Massage this spot in small, circular motions.

With your other hand start to caress her clitoris. Again, use small, circular motions, working in toward the clitoris and eventually using one fingertip to massage directly on the hood that covers the clitoris (don't touch the clitoral bud directly as most women find this too sensitive).

While you masturbate her, encourage her to play with her breasts. It'll give her extra stimulation, and is nice for you to watch.

~ TWIST ~
and SHOUT

THIS IS a little-known move that has most women dissolving with extreme joy in minutes. And you only need one hand.

The clitoris is much bigger than you imagine (think about tips of icebergs, except that we are talking hot stuff). So if you want success in this department you need to do a bit of preliminary work (and it's nice work if you can get it). Slide your first and second finger up and down her vulva, one finger on either side of her vagina. When you get to the top bring your fingertips together on top of the little hood that covers her clitoral bud. That way you will be stimulating all the nerve endings in her clitoris, and you'll be able to feel her bud swelling with each gliding movement.

When she is really aroused and swollen, moisten your thumb and index finger with a water-based lubricant or saliva. Then place them on either side of the clitoris head, and twist it gently. Start off slowly,

✳ EASY LOVER   ✳ GREAT FOR A QUICKIE
✦ NO CONTORTION REQUIRED   ⚡ NO EQUIPMENT REQUIRED

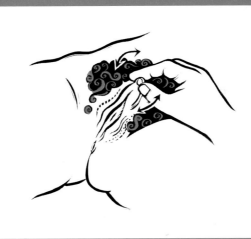

and then build to a higher level of speed and pressure. You will be able to tell by the noises she makes how fast and hard she wants it.

Some women can't bear the intensity of a lover's fingers on the clitoral bud. In this case stick to the gliding routine, and squeeze the hood rather than touching her directly. Whichever way you do it, don't stop doing it...

OOPS *Upside* ~ *Your* MAN ~

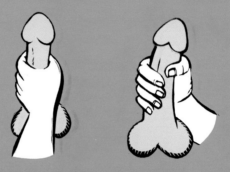

HERE'S A MOVE that will have your man in the palm of your hand. Literally. It's a sassy little hand-manipulation technique that he probably hasn't experienced before. But beware: when he has enjoyed this once, he'll want it every night.

Start by sitting in between his legs, facing him. Get comfortable—you'll want to be able to stay here for as long as he needs you. Grip his penis with your thumb at the base and the back

---

✳ YOU'LL GET THE HANG OF IT   ❋ DO IT WHILE THE DINNER'S COOKING
🐭 NO CONTORTION REQUIRED   🔩 NO EQUIPMENT REQUIRED

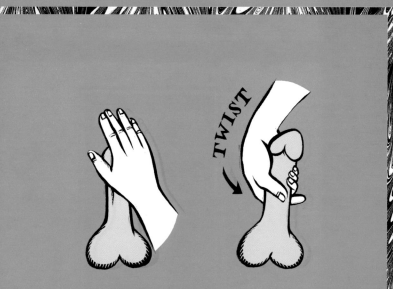

TWIST

of your hand toward you. With your fingers circling his shaft, move your hand up, slowly twisting around until you reach the top. Then release your fingers and let the palm of your hand "glide" over the head of his penis. Don't lose contact: it's the constant pressure of your hand on his penis that makes this trick work.

Then grip the shaft again—your hand will be facing the other way now, with the fingers nearest you—and slide your hand back down, twisting again as you go so you're back where you started...

Got it? It's grip, up, twist, glide, down. Sounds trickier than it is, but it's actually a very easy maneuver that'll leave him speechless.

~ STRING ~
of PEARLS

JEWELRY is not just for attracting admiring looks. One reason why it's a good idea to buy jewelry for a lady is that she can use it for lots of naughty activities. Take a string of pearls. Demure by day, they can be used to spectacular effect by night, on her and on him.

Firstly, on her. Take one end of a pearl necklace in each hand and draw the string along her vagina. The little beads tickle the clitoris, and lightly stimulate the anus. Or bundle the pearls into a handful and roll them gently over the clitoris, around and around.

On him—loop the pearls around your hand. Then use that hand to stroke up and down his penis. The beads jostle and move all over the skin, and feel fabulous.

Alternatively, a string of pearls can be used to stimulate his anus. While masturbating him, push the pearls, one by one and very gently, into his rectum (make sure that you use lots of lubricant).

✱ EASY LOVER   ✸ DO IT WHILE THE DINNER'S COOKING
🌿 NO CONTORTION REQUIRED   ▼ A FEW PROPS

Don't try to use the whole string—just four or five pearls. Then, just as he is about to come, pull the string. The pearls will press against his G-spot and heighten his orgasm.

Now you know why men love giving jewelry. And whoever said that diamonds are a girl's best friend needs to use a little bit more imagination...

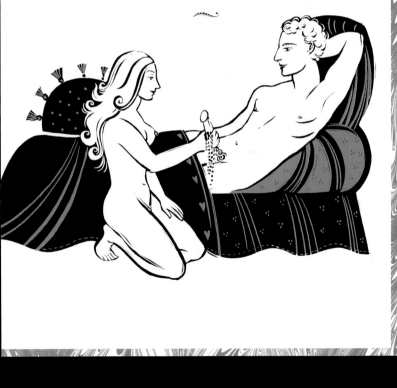

~ BASKETWEAVE ~

INVENTED BY sex guru Lou Paget, this move is a favorite among men, and women find it blissfully easy to perform.

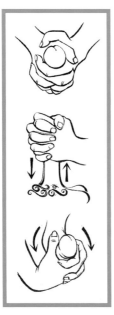

Girls, kneel down on the bed next to him and get comfortable. Then apply plenty of lubricant to the palms of both hands. Then interlock your fingers and thumbs loosely, so that they form a "basket." Slip this over his penis, so the head pokes out between your thumbs.

Then clasp your hands a little tighter around him—the idea is to form an artificial vagina with your hands—and move them up and down smoothly. As you reach the top, twist your hands. Then just continue up, twist, down, twist...

✳ EASY LOVER　　✳ GREAT FOR A QUICKIE
🐍 NO CONTORTION REQUIRED　　🔩 NO EQUIPMENT REQUIRED

As you feel him getting close to orgasm you can squeeze the shaft of his penis pretty hard, but ease off nearer the tip. The pressure of your hands, the little twist, and the feeling of all your fingers moving over him will carry him up to orgasm heaven.

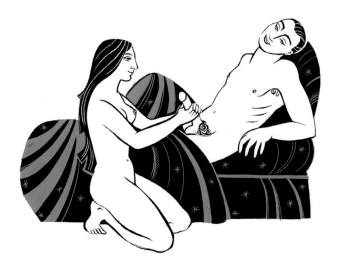

~ *The* ROLL ~

HERE'S A MOVE that's good for a penis that's beginning to flag.
It promises an erection in minutes.

Hold your hands out in front of you, palms facing each other, as
if you were going to clap. (You're not—but he'll soon give you a
round of applause.) Hold his penis between them, and roll it gently.
Imagine you were trying to start a fire. You are, really—it's the gentle
friction and heat of your palms that cause all the good feelings.

Once he has started to get hard, continue the roll but move it up
and down his shaft. Steadily increase the speed, but go careful! The
penis enjoys a degree of rough handling, but remember that it's a
delicate organ and you don't want to take things too far...

TIP: The same sort of rolling maneuver works nicely with his
testicles as well. Remember that his balls are delicate creatures and
treat them with care. Cup him in one hand and roll his balls around
gently between your fingers and thumb. Satisfaction guaranteed.

✳ EASY LOVER   ✳ GREAT FOR A QUICKIE
✺ NO CONTORTION REQUIRED   ⚡ NO EQUIPMENT REQUIRED

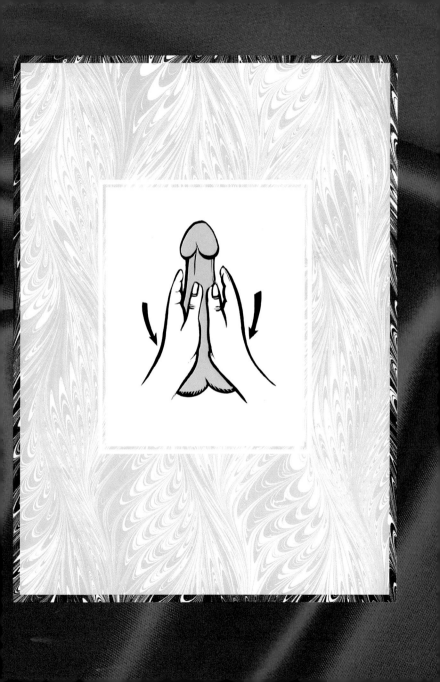

Pearl NECKLACE
~ MASTURBATION ~

ONE OF THE VERY sexiest ways to discover how the other person likes to be touched is for them to show you. It can be really sexy to masturbate in front of someone, and if they're doing it at the same time, it's even better.

This is easiest if you both lie on the bed facing each other, with your legs linked. From here you can both get a good view of each other. Then start playing with yourself in the way you like best. (Try some of the moves in this chapter.)

Girls, you can try holding your lips open with one hand and circling the clitoris with the other—he'll love the wide-open view he gets of you. If you need lubricant, have him lick your fingers and then use them to play with yourself.

Guys, holding the base of your penis with one hand will make it look bigger and fatter, as you masturbate it with the other. If things

---

✳ YOU'LL GET THE HANG OF IT   ❊ DO IT WHILE THE DINNER'S COOKING
   ☞ A LITTLE CONTORTION   ⚡ NO EQUIPMENT REQUIRED

start getting out of hand, grip hard at the base and think about football scores until you cool off a little.

Whatever you do, be sure to keep watching the other person to learn what he or she likes, and to see how turned on they become. Coming together makes this extra-steamy: it can be difficult to get the timing right, but you'll just have to practice...

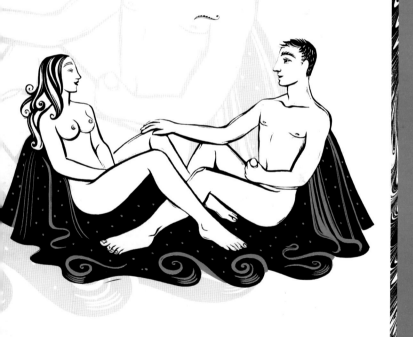

• LAP IT UP •

～ KIVIN *Method* ～

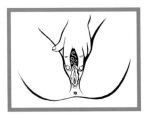

THIS BLISSFUL fast-track to orgasmic paradise is based on a Tahitian technique, and reportedly takes most women to the brink in three minutes. Plus the woman has to do nothing but lie back and enjoy. If you are really deft, and suitably dressed, you can do it with most of your clothes on.

The woman lies on her back. The man kneels or lies at right angles to her—this position gives easy access to the clitoris. He places two fingers on either side of the hood of her clitoris, then slowly runs his tongue back and forth, and over and under the hood (not the head, not yet). He begins to lick faster, at the same time using a finger from his free hand to massage the spot between her vagina and anus. As she comes, he can transfer his tonguework to the head of her clitoris. Yes, yes, yes...

❋ EASY LOVER   ❋ GREAT FOR A QUICKIE
NO CONTORTION REQUIRED   NO EQUIPMENT REQUIRED

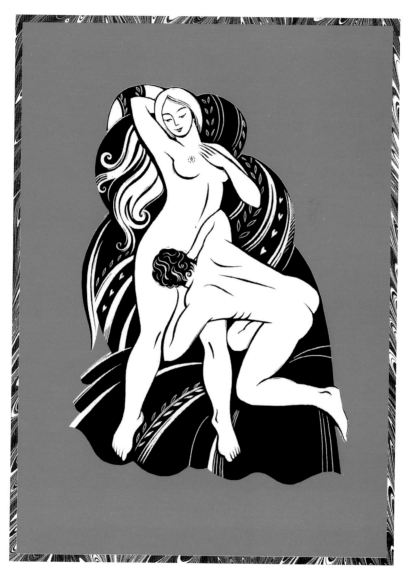

～ *Hovering* ～
BUTTERFLY

THIS IS MOST women's favorite position for receiving oral sex—and most men's favorite way to give it. Here, the woman can retain control and rest on something, while the man gets to experience the sexy pleasure of her wide open above him.

Men, lie on the bed on your back. Have your lover kneel over your face, holding on to the bed headboard or against the wall. Then, pull her down so you can reach her vulva with your mouth.

Start by placing soft, warm kisses on her clitoris and vaginal lips. When she becomes more aroused (you'll know by her lubrication—it will become thicker and there'll be a lot of it), use your fingers to draw the clitoris out of its hood. Suck on it gently, then swirl your tongue around it in clockwise moves.

Be responsive to your partner's movements. She may start rubbing her vagina along your face, signaling that she wants your

☆ YOU'LL GET THE HANG OF IT   ✿ DO IT WHILE THE DINNER'S COOKING
     ♋ A LITTLE CONTORTION   ⚱ NO EQUIPMENT REQUIRED

tongue inside her. Or she might pull away from you slightly, showing she is getting too sensitive. Listen to her body, and you'll be able to tell exactly what to do next.

TIP: In this position, you might find your mouth dries up quite quickly. If that happens, pull her down onto your mouth and use her lubrication to rewet your tongue.

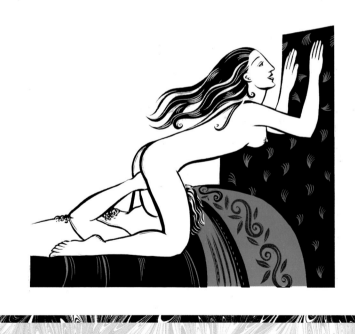

~ UPSIDE *your* HEAD ~

IS THIS WHERE the phrase "going down" originates? Maybe so. And it's one of the sexiest, most exciting ways to perform oral sex. Women adore it because they are opened up and exposed. Men appreciate the easy access it provides.

Begin by licking her vulva and pressing your tongue deep inside her vagina. Caress her breasts, and open her lips with your fingers for greater access. Hold the skin in front of her clitoris taut, and tease it with light, delicate flicks. (Don't do that for too long—it can irritate after a while.) Then hold it in your mouth and suck on it, sensuously. If you can pull and push it in and out of your mouth, she'll be very grateful. Those small, sexy moves feel wonderful.

If your partner is small and light, she can hook her legs behind your neck and you can lift her hips up off the bed. This will enhance her feeling of being exposed, but it's best to wait until the end is in sight before getting this athletic.

❄ YOU'LL GET THE HANG OF IT　❅ DO IT WHILE THE DINNER'S COOKING
♂ A LITTLE CONTORTION　♟ NO EQUIPMENT REQUIRED

When she is close to coming, hold her clitoris in your mouth and move your head from side to side, as if you were signaling "No." In fact, you'll both be saying, "Yes, yes, yes!" as the sensations spread through her body and light her fire.

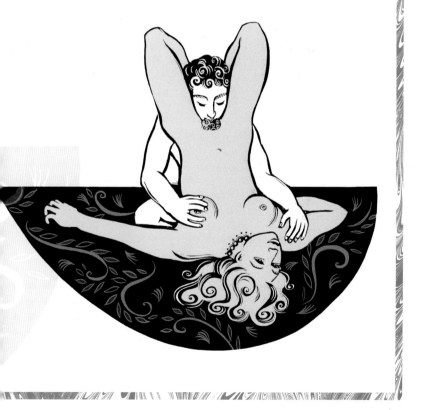

~ HUMMINGBIRD ~

HERE'S A LITTLE-KNOWN musical bedroom trick that you can perform even if you are tone deaf...

Start by giving your man a blow job. Hold his penis firmly in one hand, and slide him in and out of your mouth. Use plenty of saliva—you want your warm, wet mouth to feel as slippery and sexy as your vagina. When he's becoming very aroused, hold him quite deeply in your mouth and then start to hum. Yes, you might feel a little silly. But that's only until you see the reaction it causes: the vibrations in your mouth will pass right through his penis and stimulate every inch of him.

It's best if you hold his penis against the inside of your mouth while you hum, to produce stronger sensations. And you might want to try doing the same to his testicles: suck and grip them gently in your mouth and hum. Few women—if any—will have pleasured him in this way and it's a technique he's sure not to forget!

☆ YOU'LL GET THE HANG OF IT   ✳ GREAT FOR A QUICKIE

♪ A LITTLE CONTORTION   ♟ NO EQUIPMENT REQUIRED

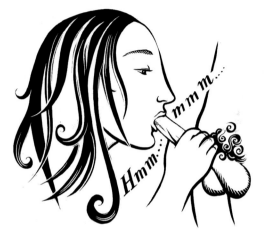

TIP: if he enjoys your orchestral performance, have him repay the favor on you. It feels fabulous if he puts his lips over your clitoris and hums, and equally good on your nipples, or earlobes, or throat. It's certainly more arousing than watching him play air guitar. Have him hum your favorite song—"I've got you under my skin" perhaps, or maybe "Ain't misbehavin'"?

ANALINGUS
~ *for* WOMEN ~

NOW FOR SOMETHING a little different. Guys, have your lover kneel on all fours on the bed. Crouch behind her between her legs, pull her hips up so her buttocks are raised, and begin licking her from behind. From this position it's hard to get the depth you're used to, but that can make it feel extra good for your partner. (There is also an "animal" edge to this position that many women love.)

Part her vagina with your fingers and lick as deeply as you can. Press your face against her, and rub one wetted fingertip over her clitoris. Then move your tongue back toward her perineum. Don't be frightened—as much as you like some gentle anal stimulation, so does she. Gently lick over her buttocks, and then use a wet finger to tease her anus. Hold her cheeks apart with your hands and flick the tip of your tongue over her anus. It'll give her a warm, wet sensation that will drive her crazy.

☼ YOU'LL GET THE HANG OF IT   ❋ DO IT WHILE THE DINNER'S COOKING
🏋 FLEX YOUR MUSCLES   🔩 NO EQUIPMENT REQUIRED

If she is really relaxed you can push the tip of your tongue into her anus. You can also use your fingers to play with her vagina and G-spot at the same time. With her lying in the same position, insert two fingers into her vagina and press down. You'll feel a small bump about two inches inside. Caress that with gentle circular motions, stimulating her clitoris with your other hand.

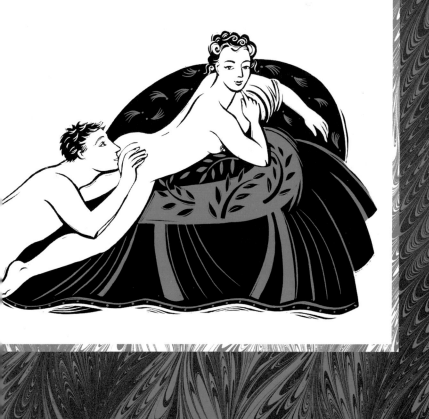

ANALINGUS
～ *for* MEN ～

THE PERFECT BLOW JOB for most men involves a little gentle anal stimulation. Most of his lovers, however, will have steered clear of this particular area. That's a bonus for you, as you'll be among the first to give him this sensuous experience.

Start by giving him a sexy blow job. In any position, use your hands and mouth to caress his penis. Covering your teeth with your lips, insert his penis into your mouth and lick and suck the length of him. Swirl your tongue over the head of his penis, and flick the tiny piece of skin that runs from his helmet to his shaft.

Meanwhile, lick your fingers and run them gently around his anus and then try pushing your finger gently inside him (you might need to use some lubricant). If he responds favorably (by raising his hips and groaning), turn him over so he is on all fours. Spread his cheeks with your hands, and slide your tongue up and down the

☀ TAKES A BIT OF PRACTICE   ❄ DO IT WHILE THE DINNER'S COOKING
💪 FLEX YOUR MUSCLES   🔩 NO EQUIPMENT REQUIRED

cleft between. Then reach around him and keep stroking his penis at the same time. If you are really dextrous you will be able to cup his balls with one hand while you run your other hand up and down his shaft (and won't he love you...).

Just as he is about to come, push your tongue into his anus as far as you can. That final added pleasure will prolong his orgasm in a way he'll never forget.

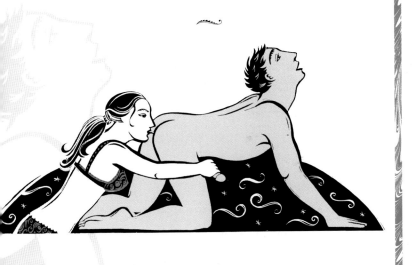

~ *How to* ~
DEEP THROAT

ADVANCED ORAL SEX for serious intimacy—this is the easiest, simplest way to use your head.

Girls, lie on your back on the bed with your head hanging slightly over the edge. Let your man push his erect penis into your mouth. At this angle, your neck is elongated and your throat is open, which means that he can slide it in very deeply. Hold his penis with one hand and guide him in and out of your mouth, licking and sucking his penis as you do. With the other hand you can massage his balls and perineum. The trick is to breathe in as his penis enters your mouth, and out as it exits. The sensations of deep penetration, and the view, will drive your lover wild, but remember guys, no thrusting.

✻ TAKES A BIT OF PRACTICE   ✻ DO IT WHILE THE DINNER'S COOKING
✺ FLEX YOUR MUSCLES   ▼ NO EQUIPMENT REQUIRED

TIP: The trick here is to relax as much as possible. You are in charge of how far he goes, and you only need a few deep strokes to cook up a storm, and then you can focus on the subtleties of pleasuring his super-sensitive tip.

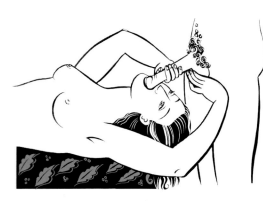

~ SIXTY-NINE ~

WANT TO KNOW the secret of good 69s? Mutual support. No, not soothing each other if it all goes wrong—instead, the kind of support you get from well-positioned pillows and a firm mattress. This sexual position is amazing and incredible—in theory. But the reality of it is all too often stiff necks and aching shoulders.

But you don't have to throw in the towel. Here's a way you can both enjoy the pleasures without the pain.

Guys, lie on your back on the bed with a firm pillow or cushion under your neck and shoulders. This will raise your head so you don't have to strain forward so much. Use your hands to pull her hips down to meet you, and don't forget that you can take a break from licking her to stroke her with your fingers.

Girls, kneel over your man so your vulva is over his face. Then slide a pillow underneath his buttocks so his penis comes up to meet you. Then just follow your instincts...

✳ TAKES A BIT OF PRACTICE   ✳ DO IT WHILE THE DINNER'S COOKING
✳ FLEX YOUR MUSCLES   ♟ A FEW PROPS

The other way is to lie on your sides facing each other, and pillow your head on your partner's inner thigh. Raise your other leg up to rest on your partner's ribcage where it's nicely out of the way. This cozy arrangement saves aching knees or back strain, and your hair stays out of the way as well.

~ VIBRATORS ~

AND WHAT TO DO WITH THEM

VIBRATORS AREN'T simply battery-powered penises. Instead, they're designed to be used outside the vagina, where their stimulation drives all the nerve endings in and around the clitoris to orgasmic heaven. Width, girth, and length aren't vital—instead, think power, volume, and portability. After all, you want to be able to use your electronic escort with discretion and enjoyment anywhere.

Recommended first-time vibrators are the small, portable battery-operated models. These get you used to what vibrators can do—namely, produce knee-trembling sensations in your clitoris—then you can graduate on to the larger, fancier novelty dildos.

Start by massaging around your clitoris with the tip of the vibrator. Try it on your breasts, your perineum, and down your vaginal lips. When you're used to it, hold it directly against your clitoris and see how quickly you orgasm. (My record is 30 seconds.)

❋ YOU'LL GET THE HANG OF IT   ✳ GREAT FOR A QUICKIE
   ♋ A LITTLE CONTORTION   ⚚ A FEW PROPS

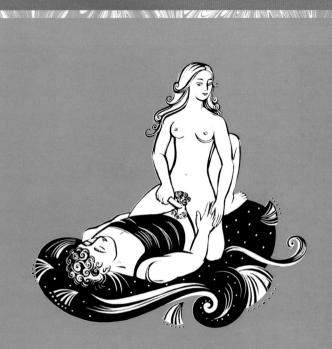

Straddle your lover, then hold the vibrator between you both so he can feel the sensations against the base of his penis as it stimulates your clitoris. (He can hold it there, too, so you can play with your breasts.) You can also try using it on him during oral sex, by holding it against his testicles, or by lubricating it and inserting just the tip into his anus when he's about to come. (Don't hold it against his penis, especially not at the tip—it's way, way too intense a feeling.)

~ FINGERTIP VIBRATORS ~

AND WHAT TO DO WITH THEM

CHECK OUT any decent sex shop or Web site and you'll find fingertip vibrators. These are awesome little toys, designed to be worn on the fingers, changing normal hands into sensory orgasm-givers. The best ones are small and neat, with a compact battery-pack that's worn on the wrist like a watch. Avoid any with long trailing wires—they get everywhere.

HOW TO USE THEM: Obviously, there are hours of fun to be had simply from a male companion strapping these on and massaging your clitoris, vulva, and breasts. In fact, make that months of fun. And, of course, you can return the favor by using them (on a lower setting—men are so delicate) while giving him a hand job. But there is a sexier option...

Have sex in the doggy-style position. Let him wear the fingertip vibrators, and reach around to massage your breasts. They are super-

❄ YOU'LL GET THE HANG OF IT   ✳ DO IT WHILE THE DINNER'S COOKING
🐾 FLEX YOUR MUSCLES   ⚘ A FEW PROPS

sensitive when they're hanging down. When you're near to coming, he can use his bionic fingertips to send you over the edge by stroking your clitoris. Incredible!

Another option: in the missionary position, you wear the fingertip toys and hold the base of his penis as he comes into you. The sensations will go right through him. The only downside is that it could well be the shortest screw you have ever had—men just can't hold back under that kind of pleasure.

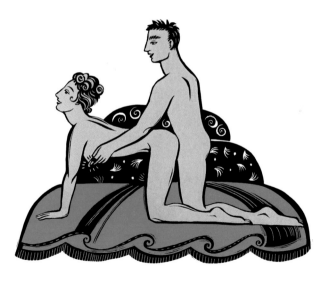

~ TEXTURED TREATS ~
AND WHAT TO DO WITH THEM

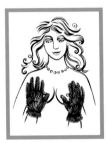

WHEN YOU WERE younger, you probably used to rub textured things over your body all the time. Children love stroking soft materials and cloths—think of a toddler sleeping with its beloved comfort blanket. But when was the last time you rubbed a silk scarf over your body? Well, if you've got any sense, it's going to be tonight!

Textured materials are the easiest sex toys to get hold of—and they're not embarrassing to buy—and they can be the sexiest to use. Collect a selection of things that feel great against your naked skin: real fur gloves; silk scarves; butter-soft chamois cloths; strings of beads or pearls; rubber gloves with ribbed fingertips; plastic car-wash mitts with chunky bristles; soft stuffed toys.

❋ EASY LOVER ❋ DO IT WHILE THE DINNER'S COOKING
♪ NO CONTORTION REQUIRED ▼ GET YOUR TOOLBOX OUT

HOW TO USE THEM: The best way is a sexy, textured massage. The receiver lies on her back on the bed with her eyes closed. Then the giver (remember, you can swap afterward) simply strokes her all over with the sensual materials. Be sure to ask what the receiver likes best—some people love the feel of real fur tickling their nipples, others adore ribbed gloves being dragged slowly up their thighs. Use the collection everywhere—on her neck, breasts or chest, hips, legs, feet, hands, and, yes, right there...

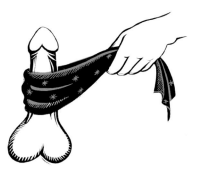

GOOD TIPS ARE: Loosely tie a silk scarf around his penis and pull it up and down. Wear fur gloves to massage her nipples and over and under her breasts. Use a very soft nail-brush to tickle and tease his inner thighs. Trail beads over her clitoris.

～ BLINDFOLDS *and* TIES ～

AND WHAT TO DO WITH THEM

IDEALLY, BLINDFOLDS and ties are used in a spirit of gentle sado-masochism. Sounds scary? It's not. It just means that you should use them to tease and torment your (actually happy) partner.

After all, they're about being denied pleasure—the pleasure of watching and the pleasure of freedom. You are not going to hurt your lover in any way. As long as you agree the rules beforehand—and are in a stable, safe relationship with plenty of mutual trust—you're free to have fun. The best blindfolds and ties are the same thing: silk scarves that can be untied quickly.

HOW TO USE THEM: The receiver is blindfolded, laid on the bed, and tied up. The easiest way is to tie both hands and both feet to the legs of the bed, so the receiver is left spread-eagled. Then begins the tease: starting at the feet, the giver kisses and licks all over the receiver's body. The thrill is that the receiver has no idea

☆ YOU'LL GET THE HANG OF IT   ❀ DO IT WHILE THE DINNER'S COOKING
🔥 FLEX YOUR MUSCLES   ⚥ A FEW PROPS

where the love assault will happen next, so be sure to keep them guessing. Girls, you can use your breasts to great effect here, massaging them all over your lover's body.

When he's close to screaming, climb on top of him and sit on his chest. Gently untie his blindfold (leaving him tied up) and masturbate yourself to orgasm. Right there, right in front of him. It's so sexy but frustrating, he'll be driven wild. Then, end his suffering by making mad, passionate love to him.

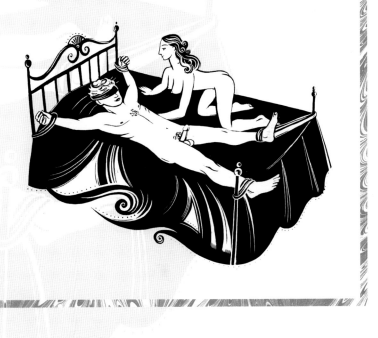

~ COCK RINGS ~

AND WHAT TO DO WITH THEM

IF YOU'VE NEVER used a cock ring, then you're missing a great trick. They work by trapping blood in the penis and testicles, giving the man a huge erection. And while they can't create what nature hasn't put there, they can help men who suffer from unreliable erections to keep going for longer.

They're for sale in sex stores and on the Internet, and are adjustable, so one size fits all. If you can buy some that are lined with soft fur, all the better. But the usual metal rings are comfortable too, and a bit more macho.

HOW TO USE THEM: While the penis is still flaccid, slip the ring over the shaft and the testicles. It should fit snugly behind the "root" of the penis. Then have your lover lick and suck you into life. You'll find that your penis becomes rock solid, because the blood isn't allowed to flow back into your body. (It's safe! Don't worry.)

✸ EASY LOVER   ✿ DO IT WHILE THE DINNER'S COOKING

🦂 NO CONTORTION REQUIRED   ⚥ A FEW PROPS

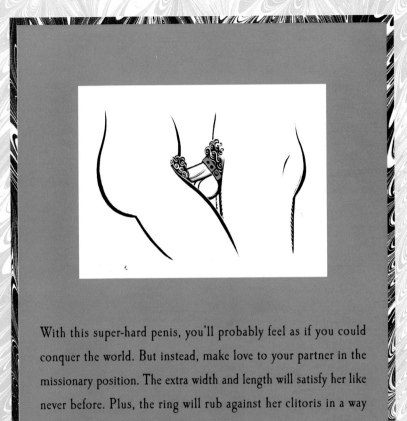

With this super-hard penis, you'll probably feel as if you could conquer the world. But instead, make love to your partner in the missionary position. The extra width and length will satisfy her like never before. Plus, the ring will rub against her clitoris in a way that she won't complain about...

After you've come, the ring will slip off easily.

~ WATER ~

AND WHAT TO DO WITH IT

WATER? That's right. It's good to drink, bathe in, and absolutely incredible in sex.

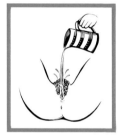

We're not just talking water beds here. Learn how to turn your bathroom into the hottest love shack around. There are several wonderful ways to come with water.

FOR WOMEN: In the tub, pour some warm water (from a pitcher or the shower) repeatedly over your clitoris. The sensations are very horny. Fill an empty shampoo bottle with warm water, and squirt it directly onto your clitoris. When it's empty, remove the lid, squeeze out all the air, and place it over your clitoris. When you let go, it'll "suck" onto you. Mmmm! In the jacuzzi, sit directly opposite a jet and feel it massage your clitoris. Take some ice cubes and rub them over your clitoris, then massage yourself until you heat up again.

✳ YOU'LL GET THE HANG OF IT   ✳ DO IT WHILE THE DINNER'S COOKING
   ✎ A LITTLE CONTORTION   🔩 A FEW PROPS

FOR MEN: Direct a showerhead over your testes and anus as you masturbate. Masturbate almost to orgasm, then dip your testicles into a cup of warm water. You'll come for longer and more intensely than usual. Insert an ice cube into your anus and masturbate as it melts.

FOR COUPLES: Take it in turns to kiss each other's genitals with mouthfuls of fizzy water. For extra fizz, apply baking soda to them first. Feel the froth. Tease each other by going down with alternate mouthfuls of hot water and cold, iced water. Use the supportive nature of water to perform more adventurous sex: standing up, with her legs around his waist, is suddenly possible.

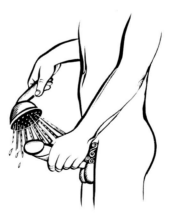

• ALL BY YOURSELF •

WOMEN

THE NO-FAIL G-SPOT TECHNIQUE

IF YOU'VE NEVER felt your G-spot before, boy are you in for a treat. It's the sexiest spot for a woman, and holds the key to multiple orgasms. Want some of that? Then here's the first step on the way to what will become a beautiful friendship.

Lie on your back with your knees bent up and your feet planted flat on the bed. With one hand, start massaging your clitoris in your favorite way. Do this for long enough to get you aroused and lubricated (but not so long that you lose control completely). When you're ready, reach inside your vagina with your other hand. Use one finger at first, and curl it back toward your stomach in a kind of beckoning motion. In this position, about two inches up inside you, you'll feel a patch of skin different to the rest—smoother and firmer. That's your G-spot.

TAKES A BIT OF PRACTICE   DO IT WHILE THE DINNER'S COOKING
NO CONTORTION REQUIRED   NO EQUIPMENT REQUIRED

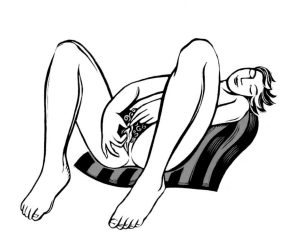

Rub it in gentle, circular motions. Don't go crazy, or the fire department will be around. Continue massaging your clitoris as you go, and let the sensations build.

You might feel an urge to urinate. Don't panic! And don't stop. It's usual when you're stimulating your G-spot. You won't pee, but you will enjoy one of the strongest orgasms you've ever known.

Have fun. And when it's all over, it will be time to do it again...

~ WOMEN ~

DOUBLE DELIGHT

AFTER THAT G-SPOT orgasm, you might be so satisfied you'd happily join a convent and never masturbate again. But we don't want that. Instead, here's a little trick that will have you moving both of your hands in ways that'll have you offering up thanks immediately.

The clitoris extends down over both your labia. So we're going to stimulate all of it. Start by planting one hand firmly over your pubic bone. Grind the heel of your hand down on it, and use those fingers to hold your lips right open. (That'll ensure you're starting to stimulate most of those clitoral nerves.)

Once the blood starts flowing and you're swollen up, begin masturbating the clitoris gently. Run your fingertip underneath the hood, very lightly tapping on the tip of your clitoris. Use loads of lubricant, and feel those waves develop. As they do, roll and squeeze the clitoris between your fingers. With the other hand, move

☀ YOU'LL GET THE HANG OF IT ❄ DO IT WHILE THE DINNER'S COOKING
➰ NO CONTORTION REQUIRED ⚡ NO EQUIPMENT REQUIRED

outward—press on the outer labia, and use the same round-and-round motion on them. Use your fingers to describe a circle all around your vaginal opening. As you feel your climax approaching, press down harder on the labia, and feel them react to the pressure. You should be masturbating your clitoris with one hand, and pressing down on your labia with the other. When you orgasm, move both hands as vigorously and quickly as you can. Bam! What a way to go.

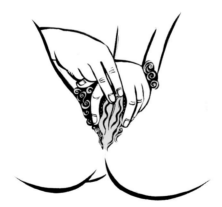

～ WOMEN ～

ALL-OVER BODY ORGASM

HAVE YOU EVER READ about women experiencing a "full-body orgasm" and get overcome with jealousy? Well, no more. In fact, you're about to become just as smug—and satisfied—as they were.

The thing to remember is that women have no refractory period—that's the space of time between orgasms where the body physically cannot come. Men have it, which explains why they keep falling asleep. But women have the physical capability to come, and come again.

But how do you do it? Really, the secret is to let yourself. I know that's not very specific, so try this—keep stimulating yourself as you orgasm, and immediately afterward. Remember, your body could orgasm for a fortnight if you let it, so let's let it!

The best way to achieve this Total Body Orgasm (because that's what these over-and-over orgasms feel like) is to use the G-spot technique described on pages 78 and 79. Use one hand to massage

TAKES A BIT OF PRACTICE DO IT WHILE THE DINNER'S COOKING NO CONTORTION REQUIRED NO EQUIPMENT REQUIRED

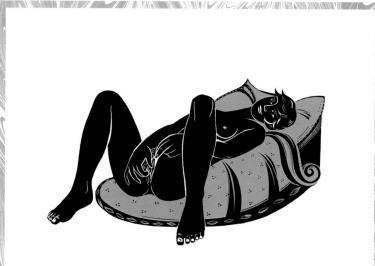

your clitoris, while the other gets to work inside you. But when you feel your orgasm approach, don't stop. Keep both hands loving on yourself. At first you might feel overly sensitive and want to stop—but don't. What you're trying to do is encourage yourself to keep coming. Over and over. No rest.

It might take a few minutes of further stimulation to start your second orgasm, but it will happen. And again, as you come—don't stop! Every orgasm you have will feel stronger and stronger until you finally (on about the third) experience the total-body tingles you've heard about. Then it'll be you who gets everyone madly jealous.

～ MEN ～

GIVE YOURSELF A BJ

IF ONLY THERE WAS a way to get a blow job whenever, wherever you wanted one. Well, there is. You can give yourself one.

OK, not literally. Every man has tried it and knows that it's just not... quite... possible. But you can get a similar sensation by using your hand and the secret weapon—lubricant. Lube will help your hand slide over your penis, and create that slight "sucking" effect on the end of your glans.

So—kneel on the bed. Apply plenty of lubricant to one hand, and begin caressing your penis. Don't touch the head—not yet—just allow your hand to glide over your shaft. Then, with the other hand, form your index and thumb into a tight ring. Grip your penis just underneath its head and turn the "ring" around. Then pull it over your penis, so it pops out. That will feel very similar to being inside a woman's mouth.

✤ YOU'LL GET THE HANG OF IT   ✳ DO IT WHILE THE DINNER'S COOKING
🦶 NO CONTORTION REQUIRED   ⚚ A FEW PROPS

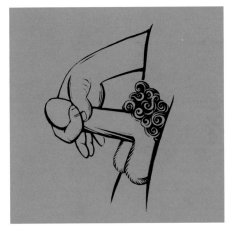

Keep massaging your shaft with one hand, and using the "ring" of your fingers with the other. Make your hands mimic a mouth, by tightening and loosening over your penis. And don't forget to massage your balls and perineum, too—as any good girl would.

When you feel yourself about to come, at the last minute, release both hands completely from your penis. Most men who've tried it says it feels "freer" and sexier, and more like the totally orgasmic release you get through oral sex.

～ MEN ～

G-SPOT WITHOUT TEARS

THE MALE G-SPOT is in an unlikely place—in your ass. But you don't have to endure an airport body search to stimulate it. Instead, here's an easy solo mission. Lie on your back with your knees drawn up to your chest, feet flat on the floor. While masturbating, use your other hand to massage your perineum—the area between your balls and your anus. Press down with two fingers and rub in circular motions. The killer spot is just behind your testicles—from here, you can reach the underneath of your G-spot (your prostate gland). You'll know when you hit the bull's-eye by the tingly sensation. Keep massaging and masturbating, then, just before you come, press your perineum firmly. Out of this world.

～

YOU'LL GET THE HANG OF IT DO IT WHILE THE DINNER'S COOKING

FLEX YOUR MUSCLES NO EQUIPMENT REQUIRED

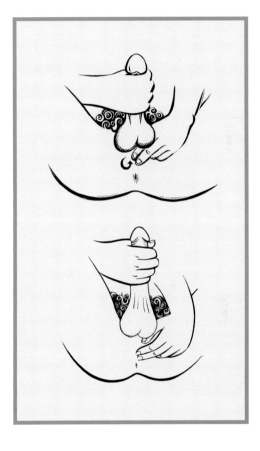

~ MEN ~

THE PROLONGED APPROACH

HAVE YOU EVER been jealous of a woman's ability to enjoy multiple orgasms? Don't be. Men can have them, too. The secret is to relax, and to STOP MASTURBATING.

Don't be alarmed, I don't mean stop masturbating forever. I mean learn when to stop during the actual act of masturbating, to prolong your orgasm when you finally let it happen.

There's such a simple way to do it. Start massaging your penis in any way you like. Play with it slowly and steadily until you feel your orgasm approach. Then—stop. If you've left it late, pull down hard on your balls, or squeeze the very base of your penis firmly, which will halt your semen in its tracks.

Then wait for the feelings to die away. After they have, start again! Begin pleasuring yourself until—uh-oh—those lovely feelings start building up once more. Again, stop. (You might need to

✳ TAKES A BIT OF PRACTICE ✳ NEEDS A SLOW HAND
🪝 NO CONTORTION REQUIRED 🔩 NO EQUIPMENT REQUIRED

squeeze a little harder this time, but you can still prevent yourself from coming.) Do this several times, and then you have permission to let go. Feel the pleasure build and just ride with it. You'll then have the longest orgasm ever—waves that just don't stop.

Just like a woman.

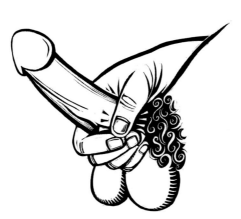

Coital ALIGNMENT
～ Technique ～

THIS POSITION is usually referred to as The Cat because eight out of ten pussies prefer it. It's based on the good old reliable missionary but soooooo much better.

The thing to remember about intercourse is that the clitoris doesn't usually get much of a look-in, which is why most girls can't come through intercourse alone. How could they? The main organ of pleasure has no stimulation at all. That's where this position comes in. It allows the base of the man's penis to rub against the clitoris—to really quite wonderful effect.

OK, so how to do it. Assume the missionary position. But then your man should pull back out of your vagina, just a little. He shifts his weight up and forward, ending with his head past your shoulders, so the base of his shaft is pressed against your clitoris. That should feel lovely already, but it gets better. Now he starts to move. But it's

✳ TAKES A BIT OF PRACTICE	✳ NEEDS A SLOW HAND
✐ A LITTLE CONTORTION	▮ NO EQUIPMENT REQUIRED

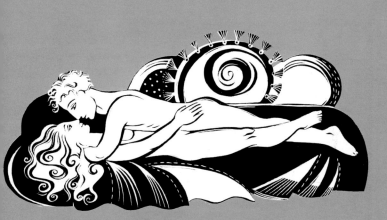

not thrusting. Oh no. Instead, he rocks forward and backward, gently, keeping his penis against your clitoris all the time. This is the best kind of "bump and grind."

At first, your man might miss his beloved thrusts. But when he feels the strong orgasms the C.A.T. can produce—and sees how satisfied it leaves you—he will come around. Truly, you will feel like the cats that got the cream.

MISSIONARY
~ *with a* TWIST ~

LET'S NOT DISMISS the missionary position out of hand. It really is a winner, and research shows it's still the most popular sexual position in the United States and Europe. But there is another way to get all its benefits while still introducing something new... Try this: the missionary position, with the woman on top.

It's very easy. The man lies on his back on the bed, the woman climbs on top of him and takes his penis inside her. Then she lies down, with her legs either between his or on either side. (It's just whatever feels best for her.) Now she's in charge, and she can thrust up and down against his penis, grind her hips around and around, or simply hold him inside her and clench her vaginal muscles.

To get optimal clitoral stimulation, thrusting against him is the best technique. He'll also like it, as he gets more depth and can feel her breasts against his chest with every stroke.

✸ EASY LOVER   ✵ DO IT WHILE THE DINNER'S COOKING
↵ NO CONTORTION REQUIRED   ▼ NO EQUIPMENT REQUIRED

Women fond of this position say it gives them the delicious feeling of being in charge, of "taking" their man. Men like it because they get to lie back and just enjoy themselves, without the responsibility of making things happen. And if buttocks are your thing, well... Its only downside is that it isn't the best way of achieving deep penetration. For that, turn the page...

ADVANCED DOGGY STYLE

~ VARIATION 1 ~

IF YOU'RE A COUPLE who love hot, deep sex, this is the move for you. You probably already love doggy style, but this is even better. It allows greater stimulation (she can rub her clitoris easily, while he caresses her breasts), and is more personal.

Start the usual way—woman on all fours on the bed, while the man inserts his penis from behind. But then you make the killer move: the man leans back on his heels, pulling the woman with him. You should end up both kneeling on the bed, with the woman sitting on the man's thighs.

Now the woman starts to slide herself up and down on his shaft. The man can hold on to her hips to direct her movements, letting her know what feels best for him. And he can also lick her spine, kiss her neck, and stroke her whole body. She can reach back and

✳ TAKES A BIT OF PRACTICE   ✳ NEEDS A SLOW HAND
🐾 FLEX YOUR MUSCLES   ❆ NO EQUIPMENT REQUIRED

caress his thighs and buttocks, or reach up and stroke his face. Because of the slight alteration in position, the Advanced Doggy is even better for hitting her G-spot: his penis will rub against it with every stroke. And he still gets that depth of penetration, and plenty of friction. Who could ask for anything more?

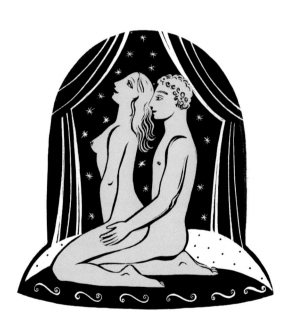

ADVANCED DOGGY STYLE

~~ VARIATION 2 ~~

HERE'S ANOTHER variation that's guaranteed to hit all the right spots. The woman is bent over the bed, with her feet on the floor. The man stands behind her. That's good in itself, but it gets even hotter when he starts his fancy footwork: for the first stroke, he pushes into her with his feet flat. Then he raises himself onto tiptoe for the second. Then back on flat for the third, up for the fourth...

The beauty of this is that his penis hits different places inside her with each stroke. When he is standing flat, he rubs against the entrance of her vagina, stimulating the clusters of nerves there. And then when he goes on tiptoe, his penis is angled to slide directly against her G-spot. It doesn't take much of that kind of action to bring a woman to orgasm. And the difference in sensations is enough to make any grown man cry with pleasure himself.

☀ TAKES A BIT OF PRACTICE   ☀ NEEDS A SLOW HAND

🔩 FLEX YOUR MUSCLES   🔩 NO EQUIPMENT REQUIRED

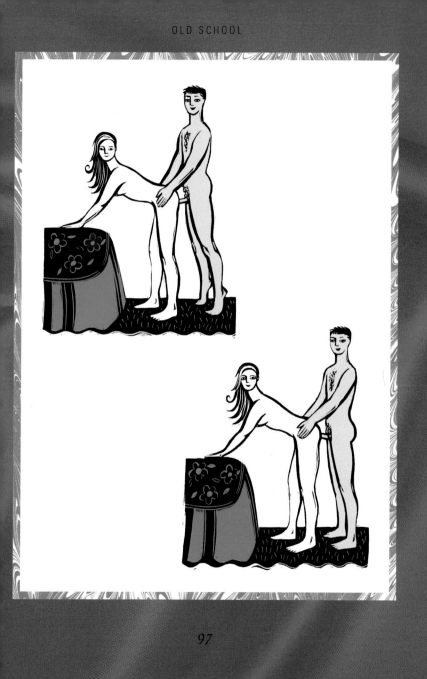

~ *The* FORK ~

LIKE SPOONS, ONLY BETTER

HAVE YOU EVER Forked before? If not, you're going to love this sexy new position. It's based on Spoons, but allows you to face your partner, so you can see just how excited they're getting, and how good in bed you are!

It sounds complicated but it's actually easy. To start, the woman lies on her left side on the bed. Then the man comes and lies down in front of her, also on his left side, but with his head at the opposite end of the bed to hers. The woman hooks her leg up over his, pulls him closer, and slides him in.

This position allows his penis to press on the outside parts of her vagina that don't usually get much action with more conventional positions. It's a new angle for him, so it takes some getting used to. It doesn't allow for much thrusting or deep penetration. But he'll soon grow to love how it stimulates the very head of his penis.

✻ YOU'LL GET THE HANG OF IT	✱ DO IT WHILE THE DINNER'S COOKING
✑ A LITTLE CONTORTION	✇ NO EQUIPMENT REQUIRED

It's also a great position for added stimulation: both partners can play with the other's feet (girls, remember how much men adore their toes being sucked), and he can easily reach her clitoris to manipulate her. She can reach his balls, and even slide her hands around his hips to play with his buttocks.

~ GIRL *on* TOP ~

VARIATION 1

GIRLS, for this position it's vital you have something to grab hold of. No, not that. But a headboard or window sill—anything to save your leg muscles from going into spasm halfway through.

What you're going to do is climb aboard your man and squat. Don't kneel astride him—plant your feet flat on the bed on either side of his hips. That's why you need something to hold on to—unless you have thigh muscles like Arnie's you won't last two minutes. Keep hold of your support with one hand and use the other to put him inside you. Then you're ready to rumble.

Holding on to the bed, or the wall, pull yourself up and down on his penis. It feels great—you have all the control you need, but you can still get the very deepest penetration. He will love it, too. In this position, he gets an incredible view of you riding his cock, and the feeling that you are really "taking" him.

❄ YOU'LL GET THE HANG OF IT   ❋ DO IT WHILE THE DINNER'S COOKING
🪶 FLEX YOUR MUSCLES   ⚘ NO EQUIPMENT REQUIRED

While you screw, rotate your hips in circular motions. This should help him hit all the places deep inside that really matter. And tease him—sometimes squatting down deeply on his penis, sometimes letting it come out almost all the way. You are truly in control here. Don't waste a moment of your power!

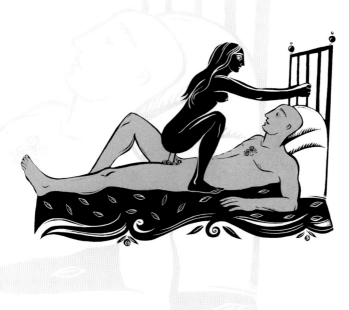

∼ GIRL *on* TOP ∼
VARIATION 2

IF THE PREVIOUS girl-on-top variation wasn't hot enough, this one is even steamier. It works particularly well if he likes your ass, because it gives him the opportunity to watch his penis sliding in and out of you, between the cheeks of your bottom.

He lies on the bed, facing up. You climb astride his hips, but facing away from him—toward his feet. Gently insert his penis inside you. You'll have to be careful—it's an unusual angle for him to be at, and his penis might spring out. Slide gently down until he is firmly inside and comfortable.

You'll immediately clock the beauty of this position: his penis presses directly against the front wall of your vagina where your G-spot resides. He is going to hit that hot spot with every move. But even so, start slowly and build up. You'll need to keep him in deep all the time to stop him from falling out, so keep your body

✳ TAKES A BIT OF PRACTICE   ✳ DO IT WHILE THE DINNER'S COOKING
✳ FLEX YOUR MUSCLES   ✇ NO EQUIPMENT REQUIRED

pressed against his. Sliding yourself along his body with every thrust, moving your hips backward and forward, is the way to go.

As his climax approaches, hold on to his feet to give yourself extra leverage. Then, when he comes, pull on his big toes. It'll prolong his orgasm and give him the ride of his life.

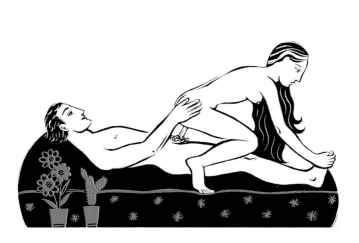

The ULTIMATE
~ MISSIONARY ~

SOME PEOPLE SAY this is better than sex. When you try it, you'll believe them. It's a simple position but it really does stimulate every part of both of you.

The woman lies on her back, facing up. The man kneels between her legs, and raises her hips off the bed by supporting her legs over his arms. Then she reaches down and inserts him.

This position lets him show off his muscular arms, as with every thrust he can pull her hips toward him. And he can see her breasts swaying with every stroke, and watch himself screw her. She has the benefit of his penis sliding directly against her G-spot.

There's no need to try to keep this up for hours on end. After a few minutes you can easily slide down together into a more conventional missionary position, but you'll have got the pulses racing and the juices flowing nicely in the meantime.

✳ YOU'LL GET THE HANG OF IT   ✻ DO IT WHILE THE DINNER'S COOKING
🦵 FLEX YOUR MUSCLES   🔩 NO EQUIPMENT REQUIRED

Alter this position to whatever angle suits you best. It's versatile—the woman can place her heels on his shoulders if his arms start to tire or you can start off with a pillow to raise her hips. But whatever you try, do try it. It's sheer sensory overload for both of you.

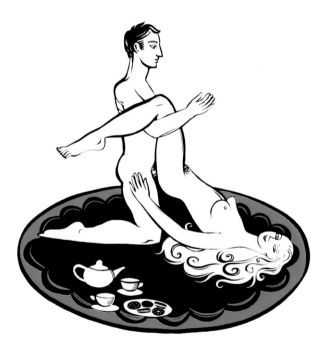

~ STAIR *Crazy* ~

NEXT TIME YOU and your lover are on the way to the bedroom, stop. If you're on the stairs, do it right there! Stairs are a fabulous aid to lovemaking. Their different heights give rise to many exciting sexual positions. And here's one of the best.

The woman stands in front of the man on the bottom step. Bending over, she pushes her hips out and supports herself on her arms. The man is behind her, standing on the floor, and—well, he can play with her buttocks, stroke her clitoris, caress her breasts, and make love to her from behind. Not bad for a night's work.

Sex in this position is good because it's adjustable: the woman can bend her knees more so she is almost lying up the stairs, giving her man a shallower screw (good for stimulating the shaft of his penis). Or she can bring her feet and hands closer together—by leaning on a stair only one higher than her feet are on—so give him a sharper, deeper angle of penetration.

☀ TAKES A BIT OF PRACTICE   ❋ DO IT WHILE THE DINNER'S COOKING
🌿 FLEX YOUR MUSCLES   ❚ NO EQUIPMENT REQUIRED

Any way is good. If the woman gets tired, the man can sit on the stairs with her sitting on his knee (with him inside her of course). Just a word of caution: use the stairs at home. They don't take kindly to this behavior in libraries.

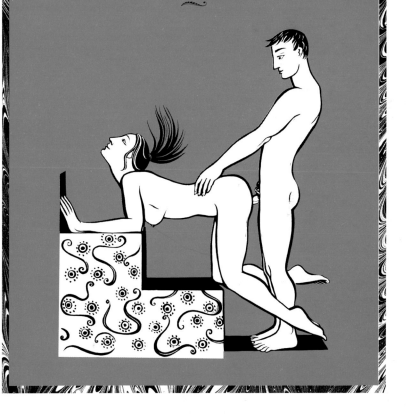

OUTDOOR
~ *Discretion* ~

YOU'RE OUT WITH your lover somewhere beautiful, and the urge just takes you. You want them—right here, right now. What do you do? Nothing. You can't. You'll be spotted. But you can take my advice for the next time you're out: wear clothes to have sex in, and you can have sex anywhere.

For this trick, the woman needs to wear a long, loose skirt. These are great, as they can be draped over the man's lap and legs and cover everything. (You also need to forget to wear any panties...)

As the man lies on his back, the woman climbs on top of him. Arranging her skirt to cover him, she can craftily unzip his pants and start massaging his penis. Then, keeping his hands under her skirt, he can insert his penis into her.

A traditional up-and-down movement will get you busted quicker than screaming, "Yes! Oh, harder, now!" so the woman should make

✳ EASY LOVER   ✳ GREAT FOR A QUICKIE
🐾 NO CONTORTION REQUIRED   🔩 NO EQUIPMENT REQUIRED

subtle forward-and-back grinds. She can also squeeze and release him with her pelvic floor muscles until he explodes. The best way is to give him three slow controlled squeezes, then three short sharp ones. That combination, along with the thrill of being outdoors, will do it every time. (Until the park ranger comes by on patrol.)

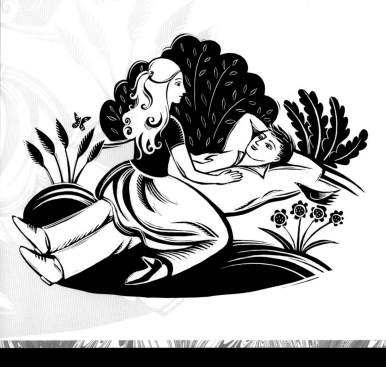

The TAKE-ANYWHERE HAND JOB *Trick*

∼ FOR MEN ∼

THIS IS A CANNY little move for giving your man a treat somewhere completely inappropriate.

Start by massaging his penis through his pants. You can get away with this in public if you stand in front of him, with your back to his chest, and use your hand behind you. Squeeze up and down his shaft, and rub his balls through his shorts.

When he's hard, unzip his pants and get his penis out of his underwear. Pull his waistband out to give room, then push his penis up, so that its head pops up above his waistband. This will stimulate the end of his penis (the waistband grips him like a hand) and gives you better access to it.

Lick your fingers and massage the head of his penis with circular, smooth strokes. Use the other hand to stroke his shaft and squeeze

---

✵ YOU'LL GET THE HANG OF IT   ✳ GREAT FOR A QUICKIE

♪ NO CONTORTION REQUIRED   ⚲ NO EQUIPMENT REQUIRED

his balls. Start working him up to a climax, squeezing him faster and harder, and using your (still wet and lubed) fingers to swirl ever more sensually over his glans.

Use a tissue when he wants to come. (It'll put him off if there's nowhere safe for him to shoot!) And then all you have to do is just wait for the compliments...

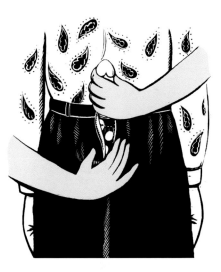

The TAKE-ANYWHERE HAND JOB *Trick*

~ FOR WOMEN ~

THIS TRICK HAS livened up many a dull evening at the theater. It's the easiest way to give a woman an orgasm when you're out in public and the movie's not what you'd hoped for.

The man places his hand on the ground (or a chair, picnic bench—wherever), his palm extended up. The woman sits on it, lightly, so that his thumb is underneath her clitoris.

Now he can use that thumb to stimulate and massage her, to get her aroused. When she is, he can push his index and middle fingers inside her. He crooks them up, so they are rubbing the front wall of her vagina. About two inches up is her G-spot—a small, smooth-feeling patch of skin—which he can massage in circular motions.

While he stimulates her G-spot, he keeps using his thumb to rub her clitoris. She can also grind herself down onto his hand,

❋ EASY LOVER   ❋ GREAT FOR A QUICKIE
🎵 NO CONTORTION REQUIRED   🍴 NO EQUIPMENT REQUIRED

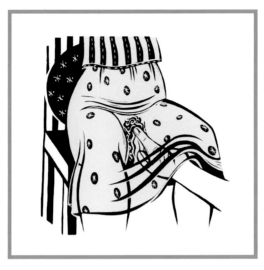

pleasuring the nerves that run all around her clitoris and vagina. And she can rock herself forward and backward, until she comes.

The take-anywhere treat she'll never forget.

UNDERWATER
~ *Love* ~

WATER CAN TURN any couple into sexual gymnasts. When you're in water, be it ocean or pool, it supports your weight, so it's the perfect venue for the trickiest sexual position—standing up.

The man stands in the water, ideally leaning his back slightly on something—the side of the pool, a rock, his yacht... The woman stands in front of him and he picks her up, holding her underneath her buttocks as she wraps her legs around his waist and mounts him.

He can then easily support her weight with his arms while she begins to make love to him. She rides up and down on his penis, then alternates with a slow grind against his stomach. This rubs her clitoris against the base of his shaft.

This is a very satisfying position for both partners, because he gets deep penetration while she has his penis press against her G-spot with every stroke.

✳ TAKES A BIT OF PRACTICE   ✳ DO IT WHILE THE DINNER'S COOKING
💪 FLEX YOUR MUSCLES   ⚑ NO EQUIPMENT REQUIRED

For more stimulation, try the same position, but this time with her facing away from him. He holds her underneath her thighs and raises her up and down on his penis. Very hot—in fact, so hot that you'll be bound to set the water boiling.

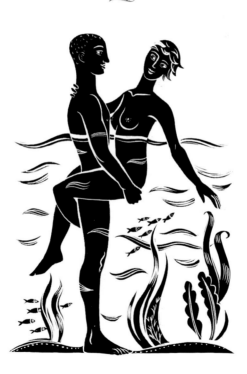

～ USE *that* ～
KITCHEN TABLE

TRY THIS NEXT TIME you're waiting for the vegetables to boil...

The woman lies on her back on the kitchen table, legs spread as wide as possible. The man stands between her knees and goes down on her. After licking her clitoris and slipping his tongue inside her, he can stimulate her with his fingers. He then enters her—keeping his weight on the floor if the table isn't as strong as it could be.

In this position, with the woman lying back, her breasts are very sensitive. He should massage them with flat, open palms as he screws her, and squeeze her nipples gently. He can also use his hands to raise her hips slightly off the table to give him a sharper angle of penetration, using his thumbs to rub her clitoris.

She, in turn, can lift her legs until her feet are flat on the table. This will give him a much deeper angle, and a better view of his cock sliding in and out.

☼ YOU'LL GET THE HANG OF IT   ❋ DO IT WHILE THE DINNER'S COOKING

     ♋ A LITTLE CONTORTION   ☗ NO EQUIPMENT REQUIRED

Keep having sexual intercourse for 25 minutes on a high heat, until done. And don't forget the various side orders that might be on hand—olive oil for drizzling, strawberries for decoration, crushed ice for refreshment. A feast of delight...

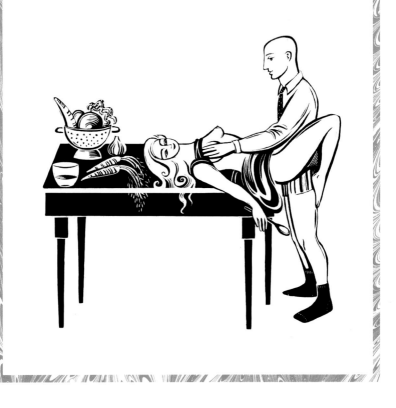

Making your OWN
NAUGHTY MOVIE

THIS IS THE ULTIMATE fantasy for most lovers—watching yourself make love on TV. But if the thought of your very private recording getting out scares you—don't put tape in the camera! Just connect it to the TV so the picture shows on the screen. That way you'll get to see everything as it happens, but nobody else ever will.

Light the bedroom with candles. They give a soft, flattering light and hide anything you don't like. Girls, wear your sexiest underwear—preferably things you can leave on during sex—and heels.

Start off by playing with each other. Give him a blow job—men adore to watch that on TV—until he's nearly ready to come, then stop. Climb on to his face and have him lick you as you watch yourself. Then you can just move downward and insert his penis into you, and have him screw you from behind—the best position to watch yourselves in.

✵ YOU'LL GET THE HANG OF IT   ✳ NEEDS A SLOW HAND

✿ A LITTLE CONTORTION   ⚑ GET YOUR TOOL KIT OUT

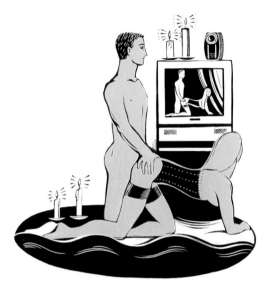

Don't get caught up looking at your body—concentrate on the sex, and watching each other's reactions. Men especially get aroused watching their partner's arousal, so don't either of you hold back.

Another do-it-yourself tip is to audio-tape a sex session. It's less incriminating than a video, but just as sexy to play back. Slip it into your partner's car stereo before he or she goes to work. Listening to that will guarantee they don't stay too late at the office.

~ S&M ~
for BEGINNERS

WE'VE ALREADY covered some very light S&M earlier in this book, with the tying up and blindfolding tips. And, for a more adventurous session, you might like to go a little further, with some gentle spanking. We're not talking full domination here. S&M is something that you should always be careful with—never try it with a brand new partner. That's not just because of safety: you have to have trust between you to be able to really let go and enjoy it.

With someone you love and trust, it can be awesome. It's a good way for a woman to regain control in sex, allowing her to be the tough one—and men can enjoy the feeling of being under her control. Or the roles can be reversed, giving the man his power aphrodisiac and the woman the delicious sensation of being "taken."

Decide first who will be the giver and who'll be the receiver. The receiver bends over a chair or the bed, and exposes their

---

✹ EASY LOVER   ❉ DO IT WHILE THE DINNER'S COOKING
   ᕫ A LITTLE CONTORTION   ⚥ A FEW PROPS

buttocks. The giver uses a cane to administer a few gentle, light strokes to the fleshier part of the cheeks. You don't need a special cane: the long, smooth, bendy sticks that support pot-plants are ideal. Don't use bamboo; it's too sharp and can break the skin.

In between spanks the giver can massage and masturbate the receiver. This can be amazingly erotic—combining sensual pleasure with the shock of pain.

FANTASY SEX

~ FOR WOMEN ~

COUNTLESS BOOKS have researched women's sexual fantasies, and most come to the same conclusion: the most common female desire is to be ravished by a strong, silent man. Sexually, it seems, conversation is nowhere. Girls just love those steely, silent types, who communicate with all-body language. So guys—become one!

Pick a night when she is expecting you. As you enter the house, take a vow of silence. Deliver strong kisses to her neck and shoulders. Silence her questions with your mouth, and reach for her breasts. While she doesn't want you to speak, she does want you to make sounds that show you're aroused. So let your desire be vocalized—groan as you undress her, moan as you kiss her breasts.

This fantasy demands that you stay in control, so don't wait for her to undress you. Instead, pull her into the bedroom and slowly, systematically undress her. Kiss and touch every part of her body as

✹ EASY LOVER   ✸ NEEDS A SLOW HAND [AT LEAST AN HOUR]
🎣 NO CONTORTION REQUIRED   ▌ NO EQUIPMENT REQUIRED

you expose it. Then, when she's naked, lie her on the bed while you stand over her and undress yourself—not taking your eyes off her for a second. Play with your penis as she watches, massaging yourself until you are rock hard. Then lean over her and kiss her—everywhere. Make sure you tease her until she is begging for you to enter her. And only then are you allowed to.

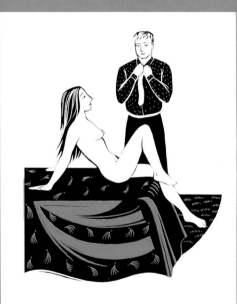

FANTASY SEX

~ FOR MEN ~

WHAT IS THE MALE number-one sexual fantasy? An insatiable woman. So the quickest way to become his number-one fantasy lover is to be that nymphomaniac girl—at least for one night.

Don't feel sexy? Then begin before you see him. Read erotica and masturbate until you almost come. Think very rude thoughts. Apply sexy make-up and change into your favorite underwear. Keep up the dirty work until he walks in. When he does, make sure you are waiting for him—ideally, just inside the door. Still wearing that sexy underwear, you should be playing with your breasts and vulva, showing him you just couldn't wait for him to get back.

Grab him, kiss him, and tell him how desperately you want him inside you. Then lead him upstairs and throw him on the bed. Grab his penis and suck it lustily, letting him know with every whimper how much you adore his cock.

✹ EASY LOVER   ✸ NEEDS A SLOW HAND
🌀 A LITTLE CONTORTION   ⚚ A FEW PROPS

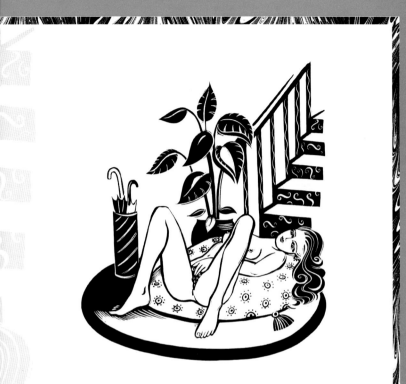

If you can pull down his shorts and climb on him while he is still mostly clothed, perfect. It'll prove even more how desperately you needed him. Then ride him as passionately as you can, and keep telling him how good it feels. If it looks like he is going to come very soon (and he probably will), slow down and grip the base of his penis firmly until his urge passes. Then start over.

∾ FURTHER READING ∾

The Best Sex You'll Ever Have, Richard Emerson (Carlton, 2002)

Come Play With Me: Games and Toys for Creative Lovers, Joan Elizabeth Lloyd (Warner Books, 1994)

The Couple's Guide to Erotic Games: Bringing Intimacy and Passion Back into Sex and Relationships, Gerald Schoenewolf (Citadel Press, 1998)

The Guide to Getting It On! (The Universe's Coolest and Most Informative Book About Sex) Paul Joannides (Goofy Foot Press, 2000)

How to Give Her Absolute Pleasure: Totally Explicit Techniques Every Woman Wants Her Man to Know, Lou Paget (Bantam Doubleday Dell Publishing, 2000)

The Multi-Orgasmic Couple: Sexual Secrets Every Couple Should Know, Mantak Chia and Douglas Abrams (HarperSanFrancisco, 2002)

The New Good Vibrations Guide to Sex, Anne Semans and Cathy Winks (Cleis Press, 1997)

The New Sensual Massage: Learn to Give Pleasure With Your Hands, Gordon Inkeles (Arcata Arts, 1998)

Pucker Up: A Hands-On Guide to Ecstatic Sex, Tristan Taormino (Regan Books, 2001)

The Ultimate Guide to Fellatio: How to Go Down on a Man and Give Him Mind-Blowing Pleasure, Violet Blue (Cleis Press, 2002)

~ WEB SITES ~

www.69sexualpositions.com—a couple's guide to 69 sexual positions and the complete Kama Sutra online

www.adultsexed.org—online sexuality resource center

www.bettydodson.com—a site is devoted to masturbation, erotic sex education, and promoting sexual diversity

www.clitical.com—site focusing on women can learn how to explore themselves sexually, and men can learn from this site, too

www.erotica-readers.com—Erotica Readers and Writers Association, erotic fiction, reviews, and links

www.goodvibes.com—sex toys, books, videos, and sex education

www.jackinworld.com—the ultimtate male masturbation resource

www.janesguide.com—Jane's guide reviews all kinds of sex-related Web sites, together with other adult-related tips and features

www.lovingyou.com—ideas to enhance your sex life

www.minou.com/adultsexuality/index.htm—Adult Sexuality Web, an online resource to help couples improve their sexual relationships and lovemaking skills

www.satinslippers.com—a Web site for women that includes erotica, fiction, sex toys, shopping, advice, and discussion

www.screammyname.com—advice and tips sex and relationships, including sex tips, new positions, and sex jokes

www.sexuality.org—Society for Human Sexuality, including library and resources on sexuality

www.siecus.org—Sexuality and Information Education Council of the U.S.

INDEX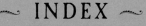